My Plant-Based Salads & Lunch Collection

50 Easy and tasty Recipes for your Lunch

Lily Mullen

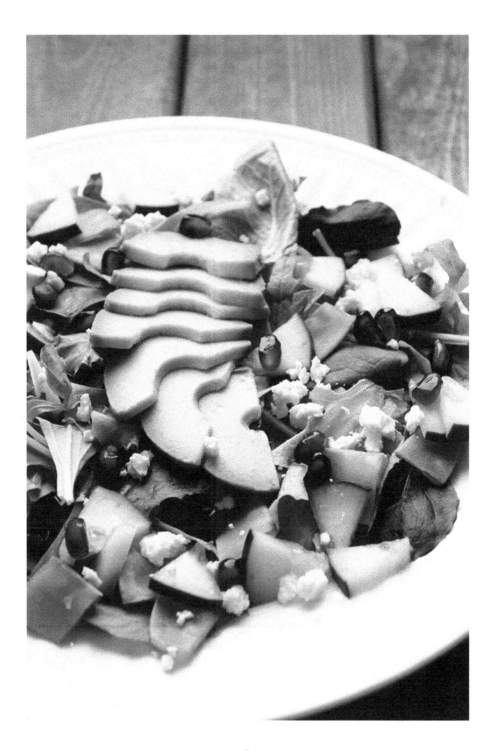

TABLE OF CONTENTS

Introduction

A plant-based eating routine backing and upgrades the entirety of this. For what reason should most of what we eat originate from the beginning?

Eating more plants is the first nourishing convention known to man to counteract and even turn around the ceaseless diseases that assault our general public.

Plants and vegetables are brimming with large scale and micronutrients that give our bodies all that we require for a sound and productive life. By eating, at any rate, two suppers stuffed with veggies consistently, and nibbling on foods grown from the ground in the middle of, the nature of your wellbeing and at last your life will improve.

The most widely recognized wellbeing worries that individuals have can be reduced by this one straightforward advance.

Things like weight, inadequate rest, awful skin, quickened maturing, irritation, physical torment, and absence of vitality would all be able to be decidedly influenced by expanding the admission of plants and characteristic nourishments.

If you're reading this book, then you're probably on a journey to get healthy because you know good health and nutrition go hand in hand.

Maybe you're looking at the plant-based diet as a solution to those love handles.

Whatever the case may be, the standard American diet millions of people eat daily is not the best way to fuel your body.

If you ask me, any other diet will already be a significant improvement. Since what you eat fuels your body, you can imagine that eating junk will make you feel just that—like junk.

I've followed the standard American diet for several years: my plate was loaded with high-fat and carbohydrate-rich foods. I know this doesn't sound like a horrible way to eat, but keep in mind that most Americans don't focus on eating healthy fats and complex carbs—we live on processed foods.

The consequences of eating foods filled with trans fats, preservatives, and mountains of sugar are fatigue, reduced mental focus, mood swings, and weight gain. To top it off, there's the issue of opening yourself up to certain diseases—some life-threatening—when you neglect paying attention to what you eat .

Chopped Kale Power Salad

Preparation time: 10 minutes

Cooking time: 40 minutes

Servings: 4

Ingredients:

For the Salad:

- 15 ounces cooked chickpeas
- 8 cups chopped kale
- 6 cups diced sweet potatoes
- 1 large avocado, pitted, diced
- 1/4 cup chopped red onion
- 2 teaspoons and 1 tablespoon olive oil, divided
- 1/4 teaspoon ground black pepper
- 3/4 teaspoons salt, divided
- 1/3 cup chopped almonds
- 1/2 of a large lemon, juiced
- 1/3 cup dried cranberries

For The Lemon Tahini Dressing:

- 1/2 cup tahini

- 1/4 teaspoon salt
- 1 lemon juiced
- 6 tablespoons warm water

Directions:

1. Place diced sweet potatoes on a sheet pan, drizzle with 2 teaspoon oil, season with ¼ teaspoon black pepper and ½ teaspoon salt and bake for 40 minutes at 375 degrees F until roasted, tossing halfway.

2. Meanwhile, place chopped kale in a bowl, drizzle with lemon juice and remaining oil, season with remaining salt, toss until combined, and massage the leaves for 1 minute.

3. Prepare the dressing and for this, place all of its ingredients in a bowl and whisk until combined.

4. Top kale salad with sweet potatoes, drizzle with tahini dressing, and serve.

Pear, Pomegranate and Roasted Butternut Squash Salad

Preparation time: 10 minutes

Cooking time: 10 minutes

Servings: 3

Ingredients:

- 1 medium butternut squash, peeled, cut into noodles
- 5 ounces of arugula
- 1 large pear, spiralized
- ¾ cup pomegranate seeds
- 2/3 teaspoon salt
- 1/3 teaspoon ground black pepper
- 3/4 cup chopped walnuts

For the Vinaigrette:

- ½ teaspoon minced garlic
- 1 teaspoon white sesame seeds
- ¼ teaspoon ground black pepper
- 1 tablespoon maple syrup
- 1 tablespoon olive oil

- 1 tablespoon soy sauce
- 1 tablespoon sesame oil
- 2 tablespoons apple cider vinegar

Directions:

1. Place butternut squash noodles on a baking sheet, spray with oil, season with salt and black pepper and roast for 10 minutes at 400 degrees F until cooked.
2. Meanwhile, prepare the vinaigrette and for this, place all its ingredients in a bowl and whisk until combined.
3. When done, place pear, walnuts, and arugula in a large bowl, then add squash, drizzle with vinaigrette and toss until combined. Serve straight away.

Black Bean Taco Salad

Preparation time: 10 minutes

Cooking time: 30 minutes

Servings: 4

Ingredients:

For the Black Beans:

- 1 1/2 cups cooked black beans
- 1/2 teaspoon garlic powder
- 1/2 teaspoon salt
- 1/2 teaspoon cayenne
- 1/2 teaspoon smoked paprika
- 2 teaspoons red chili powder
- 1 teaspoon cumin
- 1/4 cup water

For the Roasted Chickpeas:

- 1 1/2 cups cooked chickpeas
- 1/2 teaspoon salt
- 1 teaspoon red chili powder
- 1/4 teaspoon cinnamon

- 1 teaspoon cumin

For the Salad:

- 1 medium red bell pepper, cored, diced
- 1 medium head of green leaf lettuce
- 1 cup fresh corn kernels
- 2 chopped tomatoes
- 1 avocado, pitted, diced

For the Dressing:

- 1 ½ cup vegan Cumin Ranch Dressing

Directions:

1. Season chickpeas with salt, cinnamon, chili powder, and cumin, spread them in an even layer on a baking sheet and bake for 30 minutes at 400 degrees F until roasted, stirring halfway.
2. Meanwhile, prepare the black beans and for this, place them on a skillet pan, add remaining ingredients, stir until well mixed and cook for 5 minutes until warmed, set aside until required.
3. Assemble salad and for this, place all its ingredients in a bowl, toss until mixed, then add roasted chickpeas and black beans, drizzle with ranch dressing and serve.

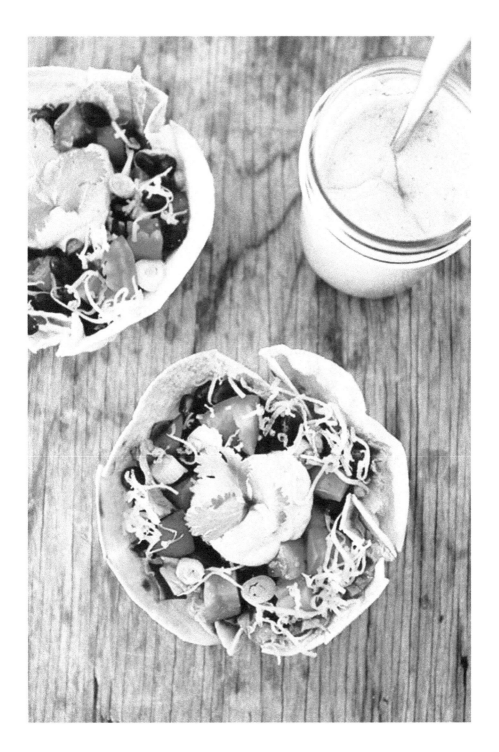

Roasted Vegetable and Quinoa Salad

Preparation time: 10 minutes

Cooking time: 25 minutes

Servings: 4

Ingredients:

For the Roasted Vegetables:

- 1 carrot, peeled, chopped
- 1 medium sweet potato, peeled, chopped
- 1 red bell pepper, cored, cubed
- 1 zucchini, peeled, cubed
- 1 tablespoon dried mixed herbs
- 1 red onion, peeled, sliced
- 1 tablespoon olive oil
- 1/2 teaspoon salt
- ¼ teaspoon ground black pepper

For the Quinoa:

- 1/2 cup frozen peas
- 1 1/2 cup cooked quinoa

- 1 cup chopped kale

For the dressing:

- 1 teaspoon minced garlic
- 1/4 teaspoon salt
- 1/4 teaspoon cinnamon
- 1/2 teaspoon ground cumin
- 3 tablespoons tahini
- 1/2 teaspoon brown rice syrup
- 2 tablespoons olive oil
- 3 tablespoons lemon juice

Directions:

1. Place all the vegetables in a large baking dish, season with salt and black pepper, sprinkle with herbs, drizzle with oil, toss until mixed, and then bake them for 25 minutes at 392 degrees F until roasted.
2. Cook the quinoa in a saucepan, add kale and peas in the last three minutes, and when done, let it stand for 10 minutes.
3. Prepare the dressing, and for this, place all of its ingredients in a blender and pulse until smooth.
4. Place everything in a large bowl, drizzle with dressing and toss until mixed.
5. Serve straight away.

Lentil Fattoush Salad

Preparation time: 10 minutes

Cooking time: 7 minutes

Servings: 2

Ingredients:

For the Salad:

- 1/3 cup green lentils, cooked
- ¼ small cucumber, chopped
- 2 stalks of celery, chopped
- 1 small radish, peeled, sliced
- 4 cups arugula
- 1 carrot, chopped
- ¼ cup dates, chopped
- 1/3 teaspoon salt
- 2 teaspoons olive oil
- 1 pita pocket, whole-wheat, chopped
- 2 tablespoons toasted sunflower seeds

For the Vinaigrette:

- 1 tablespoon Dijon mustard

- 2 tablespoons balsamic vinegar
- 1 tablespoon maple syrup
- 2 tablespoons olive oil

Directions:

1. Place pita pieces on a cookie sheet lined with parchment paper, drizzle with oil, and season with salt, toss until mixed, spread evenly, and bake for 7 minutes at 425 degrees F until golden, and when done, cool them.
2. Meanwhile, prepare the vinaigrette and for this, place all of its ingredients in a bowl and whisk until combined.
3. Add remaining ingredients in a bowl, add cooled pita chips, drizzle with vinaigrette and toss until mixed.
4. Serve straight away.

Sweet Potato Salad

Preparation time: 10 minutes

Cooking time: 35 minutes

Servings: 4

Ingredients:

- 2 large sweet potatoes, peeled,
- 1 1/2 inch cubes
- 1/3 teaspoon ground black pepper
- 1/2 teaspoon salt
- 1/2 teaspoon paprika
- 1/2 teaspoon oregano
- 1/2 teaspoon cayenne pepper
- 1 tablespoon olive oil

For the Dressing:

- 1 small bunch of chives, chopped
- 1 medium shallot, peeled, diced
- 2 spring onions, trimmed, diced
- 1 tablespoon maple syrup
- 2 teaspoons olive oil
- 3 tablespoons red wine vinegar

Directions:

1. Spread sweet potato cubes on a baking sheet, drizzle with oil, season with all the spices, toss until mixed, spread evenly, and then bake for 35 minutes at 390 degrees F until roasted.

2. Prepare the dressing and for this, place all of its ingredients in a bowl and stir until combined.

3. When sweet potatoes have roasted, let them cool for 10 minutes, then drizzle with salad dressing and serve straight away.

Butternut Squash and Kale Salad

Preparation time: 10 minutes

Cooking time: 8 minutes

Servings: 4

Ingredients:

For the Salad:

- 6 cups butternut squash, spiralized
- 5 cups kale, chopped, steamed
- 1/3 cup pumpkin seeds
- 1/2 cup pomegranate seeds

For the Dressing:

- ½ teaspoon salt
- ½ teaspoon ground black pepper
- 1/2 teaspoon cinnamon
- 1 tablespoon maple syrup
- 1/2 teaspoon mustard
- 2 tablespoons apple cider vinegar
- 3 tablespoons olive oil

Directions:

1. Place spiralized squash on a baking sheet, toss with olive oil and bake for 8 minutes at 400 degrees F until roasted.
2. When done, let squash cool for 10 minutes, then add it into a large bowl along with remaining ingredients for the salad and toss until mixed.
3. Prepare the dressing and for this, place all of its ingredients in a bowl and stir until combined.
4. Drizzle the dressing over the salad, toss until mixed, and then serve

Nectarine and Arugula Salad

Preparation time: 5 minutes

Cooking time: 15 minutes

Servings: 8

Ingredients:

- 4 cups arugula
- 2 tablespoons pine nuts, toasted
- 4 cups torn lettuce
- 3 medium nectarines, sliced
- 2 tablespoons crumbled blue cheese

For the Dressing:

- 1/8 teaspoon salt
- 1 teaspoon Dijon mustard
- 1/8 teaspoon ground black pepper
- 2 teaspoons sugar
- 2 tablespoons raspberry vinegar
- 3 tablespoons olive oil

Directions:

1. Prepare the dressing and for this, place all of its ingredients in a bowl and whisk until smooth.
2. Prepare the salad and for this, place all its ingredients in a bowl, toss until mixed, then drizzle with prepared dressing and stir until combined.
3. Serve straight away.

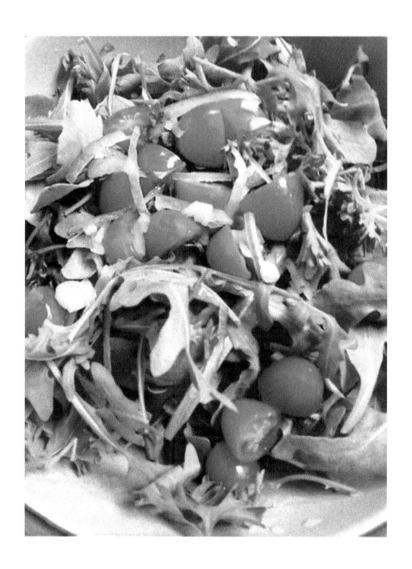

Farro, Cannellini Bean, and Pesto Salad

Preparation time: 10 minutes

Cooking time: 15 minutes

Servings: 4

Ingredients:

For the Pesto:

- 1/2 of a lemon, juiced
- 2 cups parsley
- 4 cloves of garlic, peeled
- 1/3 cup brazil nuts
- 1 teaspoon salt
- 1/4 cup nutritional yeast
- 1/2 cup olive oil

For the Salad:

- 19 ounces white kidney beans, cooked
- 2 cups farro, cooked
- 2 cups spinach
- ¼ teaspoon ground black pepper

- ¼ teaspoon salt
- 1/3 cup prepared parsley pesto
- ½ of a lemon, juiced

Directions:

1. Cook the farro until tender, add spinach in the last 5 minutes and cook until its leaves wilt.
2. Meanwhile, prepare the pesto, and for this, place all of its ingredients in a blender and pulse until smooth.
3. Transfer farro and spinach in a bowl, let it cool for 15 minutes, then add remaining ingredients for the salad, drizzle with pesto and toss until combined.
4. Serve straight away.

Chickpea and Kale Salad

Preparation time: 15 minutes

Cooking time: 0 minute

Servings: 4

Ingredients:

For the Dressing:

- 2 tablespoons olive oil
- ½ teaspoon ground black pepper
- 1 teaspoon salt
- 1/4 cup balsamic vinegar
- 2 tablespoons maple syrup

For the Salad:

- 30 ounces cooked chickpeas
- 1 1/2 bunch of kale, chopped
- 1 medium avocado, peeled, pitted, cubed
- 1/2 cup dried cranberries
- 1/2 teaspoon salt
- 1 cup diced red onion
- 1/2 cup chopped basil

- 1/2 cup almonds, roasted, salted, chopped

Directions:

1. Prepare the dressing and for this, place all of its ingredients in a bowl and whisk until smooth.
2. Place kale in a bowl, season with ¼ teaspoon salt, massage it into the kale for 1 minute until soften and set aside until.
3. Place remaining ingredients in another bowl, toss until combined, then top the mixture over kale and drizzle with the dressing.
4. Top the salad with additional almonds and serve.

Simple Quinoa Salad

Preparation time: 10 minutes

Cooking time: 0 minute

Servings: 4

Ingredients:

- 1/2 cup quinoa, cooked
- 12 black olives
- 1/4 cup cooked corn
- 1/4 cup chopped carrots
- 1 avocado, pitted, sliced
- 12 cherry tomatoes, halved
- 1/3 teaspoon salt
- 1/3 teaspoon ground black pepper
- 2 tablespoons olive oil

Directions:

1. Place all the ingredients in a bowl, and then stir until incorporated.
2. Taste the salad to adjust seasoning and serve straight away.

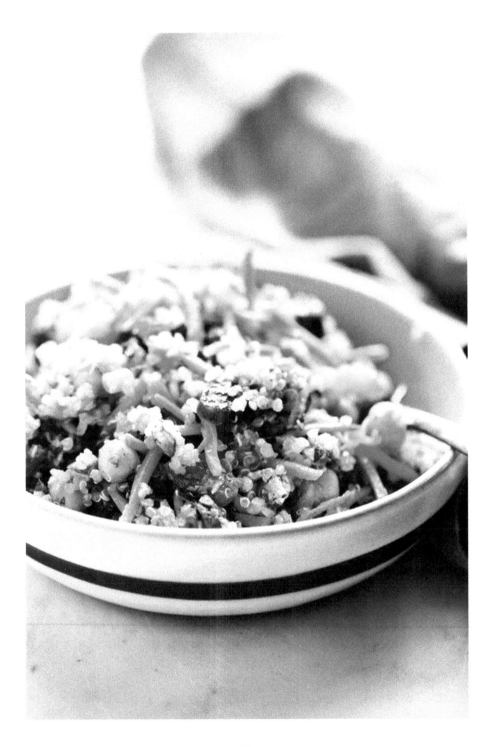

Greek Salad

Preparation time: 10 minutes

Cooking time: 0 minute

Servings: 4

Ingredients:

- 40 black olives, pitted
- ½ of medium red onion, peeled, sliced
- 4 tomatoes, sliced
- 1 medium cucumber, peeled, sliced
- 1 medium green bell pepper, cored, sliced
- ¼ cup tofu Feta cheese
- 1 tablespoon chopped oregano
- 1/3 teaspoon ground black pepper
- 1/3 teaspoon salt
- 2 tablespoons olive oil

Directions:

1. Place all the ingredients in a bowl, and then stir until incorporated.

2. Taste the salad to adjust seasoning and serve straight away.

Potato Salad with Vegan Ranch Dressing

Preparation time:2 hours and 10 minutes

Cooking time:0 minute

Servings: 2

Ingredients:

- 1/2 cup cooked corn kernels
- 14 ounces potatoes, peeled, steamed
- 12 green olives
- ½ of medium white onion, peeled, sliced
- 12 cherry tomatoes, halved
- Vegan Ranch Dressing as needed

Directions:

1. Boil potatoes for 20 minutes until softened, then let cool for 10 minutes and dice them.
2. Place diced potatoes in a bowl along with remaining ingredients and toss until well combined.

3. Let the salad refrigerate for a minimum of 2 hours and then serve

Zucchini Noodles with Avocado Sauce

Preparation time: 10 minutes

Cooking time: 0 minute

Servings: 2

Ingredients:

- 1 zucchini, spiralized into noodles
- 12 slices of cherry tomatoes

For the Dressing:

- 1 medium avocado, pitted, sliced
- 1 1/4 cup basil
- 2 tablespoons lemon juice
- 4 tablespoons pine nuts
- 1/3 cup water

Directions:

1. Prepare the dressing, and for this, place all of its ingredients in a food processor and pulse until smooth.

2. Prepare the salad and for this, place zucchini noodles and tomato in a salad bowl, drizzle with the dressing, and toss until well coated.

3. Serve straight away.

Roasted Rhubarb Salad

Preparation time: 10 minutes

Cooking time: 5 minutes Servings: 4

Ingredients:

- 8 cups mixed baby greens
- 2 cups chopped rhubarb
- ¼ cup chopped walnuts, toasted
- 2 tablespoons sugar
- ½ cup crumbled vegan goat cheese
- ¼ cup raisins

For the Dressing:

- 1 tablespoon minced shallot
- 2 tablespoons balsamic vinegar
- ¼ teaspoon ground black pepper
- 1 tablespoon olive oil
- ¼ teaspoon salt

Directions:

1. Place rhubarb in a bowl, sprinkle with sugar, let them stand for 10 minutes, then spread them in an even layer and bake for 5 minutes at 450 degrees F until softened.
2. Meanwhile, prepare the dressing and for this, place all of its ingredients in a bowl and whisk until smooth.
3. Then add mixed greens, toss until well coated, and then top with roasted rhubarb, nuts, raisins, and cheese.
4. Serve straight away.

Watermelon and Mint Salad

Preparation time: 5 minutes

Cooking time: 0 minute

Servings: 4

Ingredients:

- 5 cups watermelon, cubed
- 1 lemon, juiced
- 1 cucumber, deseeded, chopped
- ½ teaspoon ground black pepper
- 1 cup mint, chopped
- 1 tablespoon maple syrup
- 2 tablespoons olive oil

Directions:

1. Take a large bowl and place cucumber and watermelon in it.
2. Whisk together lemon juice, oil, and maple syrup until combined and then drizzle it over salad.
3. Sprinkle mint on top, toss until just mixed and serve.

Spiralized Zucchini and Carrot Salad

Preparation time: 10 minutes

Cooking time: 0 minute

Servings: 6

Ingredients:

For the Salad:

- 2 scallions, sliced
- 2 large zucchini. spiralized
- 1 red chile, sliced
- 1 large carrot, spiralized

For the Dressing:

- 1 1/2 teaspoon grated ginger
- 2 teaspoons brown sugar
- 1/4 cup lime juice
- 1 tablespoon soy sauce
- 2 tablespoons toasted peanut oil

For Toppings:

- 1/2 cup chopped peanuts, roasted
- 1/3 cup chopped cilantro

Directions:

1. Prepare the dressing and for this, place all of its ingredients in a bowl and whisk until combined.
2. Take a large bowl, place all the ingredients for the salad in it, stir until mixed, then drizzle with the dressing and toss until coated.
3. Top the salad with nuts and cilantro and then serve straight away.

Tropical Radicchio Slaw

Preparation time: 15 minutes

Cooking time: 8 minutes

Servings: 6

Ingredients:

- 2 medium heads of radicchio, quartered
- 1/4 cup chopped basil leaves
- 2 cups chopped pineapple
- 1/2 teaspoon ground black pepper
- 1/2 teaspoon salt
- 2 tablespoons olive oil
- 2 tablespoons orange juice

Directions:

1. Brush radicchio with oil on both sides and then grill for 8 minutes until tender, turning halfway.
2. When grilled, let radicchio cool for 10 minutes, then slice them thinly and place them in a bowl.
3. Add remaining ingredients, toss until combined, and serve.

Carrot Salad with Quinoa

Preparation time: 10 minutes

Cooking time: 0 minute

Servings: 6

Ingredients:

For the Salad:

- 1 cup quinoa, cooked
- 3 cups grated carrots
- 3 scallions, sliced
- 2 cups sliced celery
- 1 bunch of cilantro, chopped
- ½ teaspoon minced garlic
- ½ teaspoon salt
- ½ teaspoon allspice
- ¼ teaspoon ground black pepper
- 1 tablespoon apple cider vinegar
- ½ teaspoon cayenne pepper
- ½ cup chopped almonds, toasted

For the Vinaigrette:

- ½ teaspoon salt
- 2 tablespoons honey
- ½ teaspoon ground black pepper
- ¼ cup olive oil
- ¼ cup apple cider vinegar

Directions:

1. Prepare the vinaigrette and for this, place all of its ingredients in a bowl and whisk until combined.
2. Prepare the salad and for this, place all of its ingredients in a bowl, drizzle with the vinaigrette, and toss until well combined.
3. Serve straight away.

Kohlrabi Slaw

Preparation time: 10 minutes

Cooking time: 0 minute

Servings: 4

Ingredients:

For the Citrus Dressing:

- 1/2 teaspoon salt
- 1/4 cup honey
- 1 tablespoon rice wine vinegar
- ¼ cup of orange juice
- 2 tablespoons lime juice
- 1/4 cup olive oil

For the Salad:

- 6 cups kohlrabi, trimmed, peeled, cut into matchsticks
- ½ of a jalapeno, minced
- 1 orange, juiced, zested
- ½ cup chopped cilantro
- 1 lime, juiced, zested
- 1/4 cup chopped scallion

Directions:

1. Prepare the dressing and for this, place all of its ingredients in a small bowl and whisk until smooth.
2. Take a large bowl, place all the ingredients for the salad in it, top with prepared dressing and toss until well coated.
3. Top the salad with almonds and then serve straight away

Fennel Salad with Cucumber and Dill

Preparation time: 20 minutes

Cooking time: 0 minute

Servings: 4

Ingredients:

- 2 large fennel bulbs, cored, trimmed, cored, shaved into thin slices
- 3 small cucumbers, shaved into thin sliced
- 1/2 cup chopped dill
- 1/4 cup sliced white onion,
- 1/3 teaspoon salt
- 1/3 teaspoon ground black pepper
- 1/3 cup olive oil
- ¼ cup lemon juice

Directions:

1. Take a large bowl, place all the ingredients in it, and toss until well coated.

2. Let the salad refrigerate for 15 minutes and then serve.

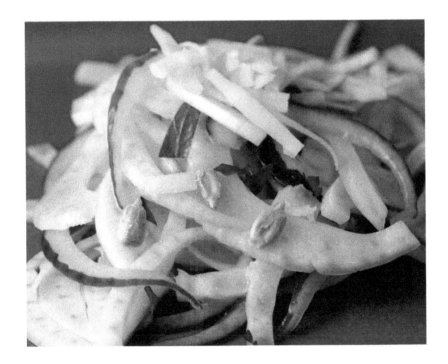

Lemon, Basil and Orzo Salad

Preparation time: 10 minutes

Cooking time: 0 minute

Servings: 4

Ingredients:

For the Salad:

- 1 cup orzo pasta, cooked
- 2 cups sliced cucumbers
- 1 cup cherry tomatoes, halved
- 1 cup baby arugula

For the Dressing:

- 2 cloves of garlic, peeled
- 1 lemon, zested
- 1 cup basil
- 1/3 cup olive oil
- ¼ teaspoon ground black pepper
- ½ teaspoon salt
- 2 tablespoons lemon juice

Directions:

1. Prepare the dressing, and for this, place all of its ingredients in a food processor and pulse until smooth.
2. Take a large bowl, place orzo pasta in it, add prepared dressing in it, toss until mixed, then add remaining ingredients for the salad in it and toss until just mixed.
3. Serve straight away.

Kale Slaw

Preparation time: 10 minutes

Cooking time: 0 minute

Servings: 4

Ingredients:

For the Salad:

- ½ small head of cabbage, shredded
- ¼ cup mixed herbs
- ¼ of a medium red onion, peeled, sliced
- 1 small bunch of kale, cut into ribbons

For the Dressing:

- 1 teaspoon minced garlic
- ¼ teaspoon ground black pepper
- ¼ teaspoon salt
- ¼ teaspoon red chili flakes
- ¼ cup olive oil
- 1 lemon, juiced

For the Topping:

- 1 teaspoon hemp seeds

- 1 teaspoon sunflower
- 1 teaspoon pumpkin seeds

Directions:

1. Prepare the dressing and for this, place all of its ingredients in a small bowl and whisk until smooth.
2. Take a large bowl, place all the ingredients for the salad in it, top with prepared dressing and toss until well coated.
3. Garnish the salad with all the seeds and then serve.

Carrot Salad with Cashews

Preparation time: 20 minutes

Cooking time: 0 minute

Servings: 4

Ingredients:

- 4 cups grated carrots
- 3 scallions, chopped
- ½ cup cilantro, chopped
- ½ teaspoon minced garlic
- 1 teaspoon minced ginger
- ½ teaspoon salt
- ¼ teaspoon cayenne pepper
- ¼ teaspoon ground black pepper
- 1 teaspoon curry powder
- 2 tablespoons honey
- ½ teaspoon ground turmeric
- 1/3 cup raisins
- ½ cup toasted cashews
- 1 tablespoon orange zest
- 3 tablespoon lime juice

- 1/4 cup olive oil

Directions:

1. Take a large bowl, place all the ingredients in it, and toss until well coated.
2. Let the salad refrigerate for 15 minutes and then serve.

Butternut Squash Soup

Preparation Time: 15 minutes

Cooking Time: 25 minutes

Servings: 6

Ingredients:

- 2 tbsp olive oil
- 1 cup onion, chopped
- 1 cup cilantro
- 1 ginger, sliced thinly
- 2 cups pears, chopped
- ½ tsp ground coriander
- Salt to taste
- 2 ½ lb. butternut squash, cubed
- 1 tsp. lime zest
- 26 oz. coconut milk
- 1 tbsp. lime juice
- ½ cup plain yogurt

Directions:

1. Pour the oil into a pan over medium heat.
2. Add the onion, cilantro, ginger, pears, coriander and salt.
3. Stir and cook for 5 minutes.
4. Transfer to a pressure cooker.
5. Stir in the squash and lime zest.
6. Pour in the coconut milk.
7. Cook on high for 20 minutes.
8. Release pressure naturally.
9. Stir in the lime juice.
10. Transfer to a blender.
11. Pulse until smooth.
12. Reheat and stir in yogurt before serving.

Tomato Soup with Kale & White Beans

Preparation Time: 5 minutes

Cooking Time: 7 minutes

Servings: 4

Ingredients:

- 28 oz. tomato soup
- 1 tbsp. olive oil
- 3 cups kale, chopped
- 14 oz. cannellini beans, rinsed and drained
- 1 tsp. garlic, crushed and minced
- ¼ cup Parmesan cheese, grated

Directions:

1. Pour the soup into a pan over medium heat.
2. Add the oil and cook the kale for 2 minutes.
3. Stir in the beans and garlic.
4. Simmer for 5 minutes.
5. Sprinkle with Parmesan cheese before serving.

Yummy Lentil Rice Soup

Servings: 6

Preparation time: 4 hours and 15 minutes

Ingredients:

- 2 cups of brown rice, uncooked
- 2 cups of lentils, uncooked
- 1/2 cup of chopped celery
- 1 cup of chopped carrots
- 1 cup of sliced mushrooms
- 1/2 of a medium-sized white onion, peeled and chopped
- 1 teaspoon of minced garlic
- 1 tablespoon of salt
- 1/2 teaspoon of ground black pepper
- 1 cup of vegetable broth
- 8 cups of water

Directions:

1. Using a 6-quarts slow cooker, place all the ingredients except for mushrooms and stir until it mixes properly.

2. Cover with lid, plug in the slow cooker and let it cook for 3 to 4 hours at the high setting or until it is cooked thoroughly.

3. Pour in the mushrooms, stir and continue cooking for 1 hour at the low heat setting or until it is done.

4. Serve right away.

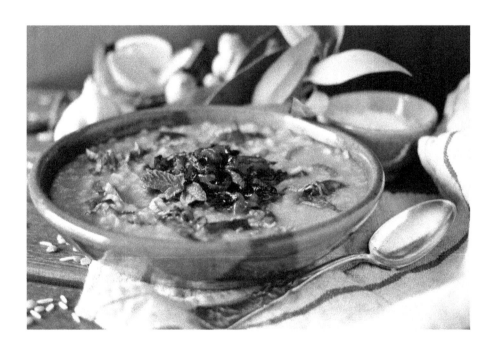

Black Bean & Corn Salad with Avocado

Total Preparation & Cooking time: 20 mins.

Servings: 6

Ingredients:

- 1 and 1⁄2 cups corn kernels, cooked & frozen or canned
- 1⁄2 cup olive oil
- 1 minced clove garlic
- 1⁄3 cup lime juice, fresh
- 1 avocado (peeled, pitted & diced)
- 1⁄8 tsp. cayenne pepper
- 2 cans black beans, (approximately 15 oz.)
- 6 thinly sliced green onions
- 1⁄2 cup chopped cilantro, fresh
- 2 chopped tomatoes
- 1 chopped red bell pepper
- Chili powder 1⁄2 tsp. salt

Directions:

1. In a small jar, place the olive oil, lime juice, garlic, cayenne, and salt.
2. Cover with lid; shake until all the ingredients under the jar are mixed well.
3. Toss the green onions, corn, beans, bell pepper, avocado, tomatoes, and cilantro together in a large bowl or plastic container with a cover.
4. Shake the lime dressing for a second time and transfer it over the salad ingredients.
5. Stir salad to coat the beans and vegetables with the dressing; cover & refrigerate.
6. To blend the flavors completely, let this sit a moment or two.
7. Remove the container from the refrigerator from time to time; turn upside down & back gently a couple of times to reorganize the dressing.

Edamame Salad

Serves: 1

Preparation Time: 15 Minutes

Ingredients:

- ¼ Cup Red Onion, Chopped
- 1 Cup Corn Kernels, Fresh
- 1 Cup Edamame Beans, Shelled & Thawed
- 1 Red Bell Pepper, Chopped
- 2-3 Tablespoons Lime Juice, Fresh
- 5-6 Basil Leaves, Fresh & Sliced
- 5-6 Mint Leaves, Fresh & Sliced
- Sea Salt & Black Pepper to Taste

Directions:

1. Place everything into a Mason jar, and then seal the jar tightly.
2. Shake well before serving.

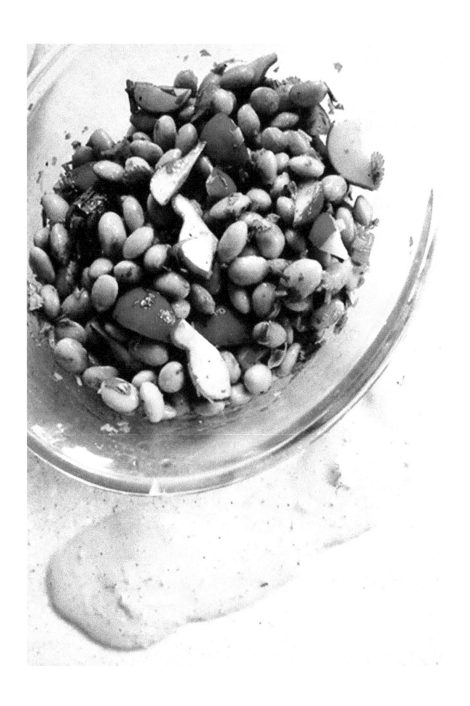

Olive & Fennel Salad

Serves: 3

Preparation Time: 5 Minutes

Ingredients:

- 6 Tablespoons Olive Oil
- 3 Fennel Bulbs, Trimmed, Cored & Quartered
- 2 Tablespoons Parsley, Fresh & Chopped
- 1 Lemon, Juiced & Zested
- 12 Black Olives
- Sea Salt & Black Pepper to Taste

Directions:

1. Grease your baking dish, and then place your fennel in it.
2. Make sure the cut side is up.
3. Mix your lemon zest, lemon juice, salt, pepper and oil, pouring it over your fennel.
4. Sprinkle your olives over it, and bake at 400.
5. Serve with parsley.

Zucchini & Lemon Salad

Serves: 2

Preparation Time: 3 Hours 10 Minutes

Ingredients:

- 1 Green Zucchini, Sliced into Rounds
- 1 Yellow Squash, Zucchini, Sliced into Rounds
- 1 Clove Garlic, Peeled & Chopped
- 2 Tablespoons Olive Oil
- 2 Tablespoons Basil, Fresh
- 1 Lemon, Juiced & Zested
- ¼ Cup Coconut Milk
- Sea Salt & Black Pepper to Taste

Directions:

1. Refrigerate all ingredients for three hours before serving. Interesting Facts: Lemons are popularly known as harboring loads of Vitamin C, but are also excellent sources of folate, fiber, and antioxidants.
2. Bonus: Helps lower cholesterol.

3. Double Bonus: Reduces risk of cancer and high blood pressure.

Hearty Vegetarian Lasagna Soup

Servings: 10

Preparation time: 7 hours and 20 minutes

Ingredients:

- 12 ounces of lasagna noodles
- 4 cups of spinach leaves
- 2 cups of brown mushrooms, sliced
- 2 medium-sized zucchinis, stemmed and sliced
- 28 ounce of crushed tomatoes
- 1 medium-sized white onion, peeled and diced
- 2 teaspoon of minced garlic
- 1 tablespoon of dried basil
- 2 bay leaves
- 2 teaspoons of salt
- 1/8 teaspoon of red pepper flakes
- 2 teaspoons of ground black pepper
- 2 teaspoons of dried oregano
- 15-ounce of tomato sauce
- 6 cups of vegetable broth

Directions:

1. Grease a 6-quarts slow cooker and place all the ingredients in it except for the lasagna and spinach.
2. Cover the top, plug in the slow cooker; adjust the cooking time to 7 hours and let it cook on the low heat setting or until it is properly done.
3. In the meantime, cook the lasagna noodles in the boiling water for 7 to 10 minutes or until it gets soft.
4. Then drain and set it aside until the slow cooker is done cooking.
5. When it is done, add the lasagna noodles into the soup along with the spinach and continue cooking for 10 to 15 minutes or until the spinach leaves wilts.
6. Using a ladle, serving it in a bowl.

Spicy mustard

Preparation Time: 20minutes

Ingredients:

- 1 teaspoon of red wine vinegar
- ¼ teaspoon of cayenne pepper
- ⅛ teaspoon of chili powder

Directions:

1. Mix and mix all INGREDIENTS in a small bowl.
2. Save up to 1 week (maybe more time, but I haven't tried it).
3. Try adding more INGREDIENTS to your liking

Lemon Mustard Baby Veggies

Preparation Time: 15 minutes

Cooking Time: 10 minutes

Servings: 8

Ingredients:

- 1 clove garlic, minced
- 2 tablespoons fresh lemon juice
- 1 teaspoon Dijon mustard
- 2 tablespoons olive oil, divided
- 2 tablespoons water
- ½ teaspoon lemon zest
- 2 teaspoons fresh basil, chopped
- 1 lb. baby zucchini
- ½ lb. baby carrots
- ½ lb. baby potatoes
- 12 cherry tomatoes

Directions:

1. Mix garlic, lemon juice, mustard, half of olive oil, water and lemon zest in a bowl.
2. Transfer to a glass jar with lid.
3. Pour remaining olive oil in a pan over medium heat.
4. Once hot, add the vegetables.
5. Cook until tender.
6. Drain and transfer in a food container.
7. When ready to eat, reheat veggies and toss in the lemon mustard sauce.

Roasted Root Vegetables

Preparation Time: 20 minutes

Cooking Time: 1 hour and 10 minutes

Servings: 8

Ingredients:

- 2 cups celery root, sliced
- 1 ½ cups baby carrots, peeled
- 8 oz. baby potatoes, sliced in half
- 3 parsnips, sliced
- 1 fennel bulb, cored and quartered
- 2 shallots, sliced
- 2 tablespoons olive oil
- Salt and pepper to taste

Directions:

1. Preheat your oven to 325 degrees F.
2. In a baking pan, put all the root vegetables and toss to combine.
3. Drizzle with oil and season with salt and pepper.
4. Mix well.

5. Bake for 1 hour.

6. Increase temperature of your oven to 425 degrees F.

7. Bake for 10 minutes.

8. Transfer to a food container.

9. Reheat in pan without oil before serving.

Broccoli & Cauliflower in Lemon-Dill Sauce

Preparation Time: 10 minutes

Cooking Time: 20 minutes

Servings: 4

Ingredients:

- 1 tablespoon olive oil
- 2 teaspoons lemon juice
- ½ teaspoon dried dill weed
- 1 clove garlic, minced
- Salt and pepper to taste
- ⅛ teaspoon dry mustard
- 2 cups cauliflower florets
- 2 cups broccoli florets
- Fresh dill sprigs

Directions:

1. Preheat your oven to 375 degrees F.

2. Add olive oil, lemon juice, dill, garlic, salt, pepper and mustard in a glass jar with lid.
3. Shake to blend well.
4. In a baking pan, toss cauliflower and broccoli in 3 tablespoons lemon dill sauce.
5. Bake in the oven for 20 minutes or until tender.
6. Toss in the remaining sauce before serving.

Sun-drenched tomato SPREAD

Preparation Time: 30minutes

Ingredients:

- 1 cup raw yarn
- 1 cup sun-dried tomatoes (not oil-packed!)
- 1/2 cup water
- 2 garlic cloves
- 2 green onions
- 4-5 large fresh basil leaves
- Juice of 1/2 lemon
- 1/2 tsp salt
- Pepper

Directions:

1. Soak the cucumber and sun-dried tomatoes in hot water for 30 minutes.
2. Rinse and rinse.
3. Place the licorice and sun-dried tomatoes in a food processor that fits into the S blade.
4. Start the puree, then pour 1/2 cup into the water.

5. Pour the puree over the sides of the bowl until smooth.
6. Add remaining INGREDIENTS and puree until smooth.
7. Get into the fridge

Spicy marinara sauce

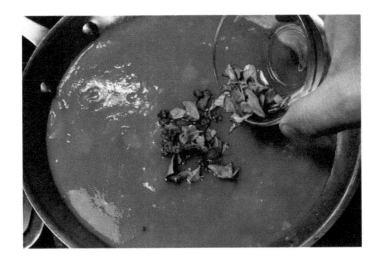

Preparation Time: 30minutes

Ingredients:

- 1/2 sweet onion (dough)
- 1/4 cup vegetable broth (or water) (extra 1-2 tbsp, if needed)
- 3 garlic cloves (minced)
- 1 4-1 2 tsp crushed red pepper flakes
- 28 ounces canned crushed tomatoes
- 1/2 tsp salt (or to taste)
- 2 tsp dried basil
- 1 tsp dried oregano
- 1 teaspoon balsamic vinegar

Directions:

1. Dried onions in vegetable broth (or water) for 4-5 minutes until softened.
2. If the onion starts to stick, add an additional 1-2 tbsp vegetable broth (or water).
3. Add grated garlic and red pepper flakes and sauce for 1 minute.
4. Using a blender, blend the sauce until smooth (or desired consistency).
5. Alternatively, you can carefully slice the sauce into a blender, puree.
6. Taste and adjust seasoning as needed.
7. Enjoy

Maple Walnut Vegan Cream Cheese

Preparation Time: 30minutes

Ingredients:

- 1 1/2 cup raw yarn (soaked in water for several hours or overnight)
- 1/4 cup dairy free plain yogurt (I used tasty coconut downstairs)
- 4 tbsp pure maple syrup
- 2 tbsp fresh lemon juice
- 1/2 tsp salt (I used Himalayan pink salt)
- 1/4 cup finely chopped walnuts

Directions:

1. Make sure your kelps have been soaked in water for at least 3-4 hours or overnight. The longer the better.
2. In a food processor bowl, clean the soaked licorice, yogurt, maple syrup, lemon juice and salt.

Directions:

1. Rinse sides as needed so that all INGREDIENTS are incorporated.
2. Continue cleaning until the mixture is silky smooth.
3. Transfer the mixture to a small bowl.
4. Sprinkle with chopped walnuts.
5. Store in refrigerator.

Cauliflower & Apple Salad

Serves: 4 Time: 25 Minutes

Calories: 198 | Protein: 7 | Grams Fat: 8 Grams | Carbs: 32 Grams

Ingredients:

- 3 Cups Cauliflower, Chopped into Florets
- 2 Cups Baby Kale
- 1 Sweet Apple, Cored & Chopped
- ¼ Cup Basil, Fresh & Chopped
- ¼ Cup Mint, Fresh & Chopped
- ¼ Cup Parsley, Fresh & Chopped
- 1/3 Cup Scallions, Sliced Thin
- 2 Tablespoons Yellow Raisins
- 1 Tablespoon Sun Dried Tomatoes, Chopped
- ½ Cup Miso Dressing, Optional
- ¼ Cup Roasted Pumpkin Seeds, Optional

Directions:

1. Combine everything together, tossing before serving.

Interesting Facts:

This vegetable is an extremely high source of vitamin A, vitamin B1, B2 and B3.

Spinach & Orange Salad

Serves: 6

Time: 15 Minutes

Calories: 99 | Protein: 2.5 Grams | Fat: 5 Grams | Carbs: 13.1 Grams

Ingredients:

- ¼-1/3 Cup Vegan Dressing
- 3 Oranges, Medium, Peeled, Seeded & Sectioned
- ¾ lb. Spinach, Fresh & Torn
- 1 Red Onion, Medium, Sliced & Separated into Rings

Directions:

1. Toss everything together, and serve with dressing.

Interesting Facts:

Spinach is one of the most superb green veggies out there. Each serving is packed with 3 grams of protein and is a highly encouraged component of the plant-based diet.

Mushroom Pasta

Preparation time: 10 minutes

Cooking time: 30 minutes

Servings: 4

Ingredients:

- 1 Cup Coconut Milk
- 1 ½ Cups Mushrooms, Sliced
- 1 Teaspoon Arrowroot
- 1 Cup Pasta
- 2 Cups Water

Directions:

2. Press sauté and then pour in a little bit of your coconut milk, adding in your mushrooms.
3. Cook for three minutes, and then stir in your pasta, water and the remaining milk.
4. Secure the lid, and then cook on high pressure for seven minutes.
5. Use a quick release, and then press sauté again.

6. Whisk in our arrowroot powder, allowing it to simmer until it thickens.

7. Serve warm once thickened.

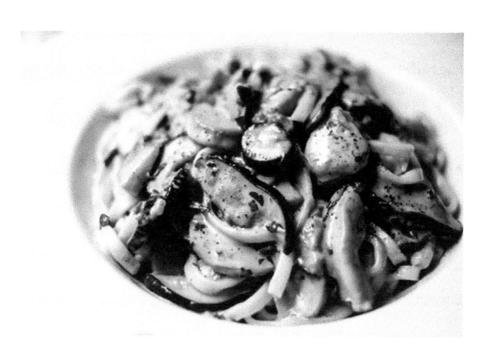

Gobi Masala

Preparation time: 10 minutes

Cooking time: 30 minutes

Servings: 4

Ingredients:

- 1 Clove Garlic, Minced
- 1 White Onion, Diced
- 1 Teaspoon Cumin Seeds
- 1 Tablespoons olive Oil
- 1 Head Cauliflower, Chopped
- 1 Teaspoon Cumin
- 1 Tablespoon Coriander
- ½ Teaspoon Sea Salt, Fine
- 1 Cup Water
- ½ Teaspoon Garam Masala Cooked Rice to Serve

Directions:

1. Put your instant pot on sauté and press low, and then add the oil in.

2. once it's hot cook your cumin seeds for thirty seconds, and stir often to keep it from burning.
3. Add the onion in, cooking for another three minutes.
4. Keep stirring to keep it from burning.
5. Add in the garlic, cooking for another half a minute.
6. Add the coriander, cauliflower, cumin, garam masala, water and salt.
7. Lock your lid and cook on high pressure for one minute.
8. Use a quick release, and serve over rice.

Vegan Hoppin' Rice Salad

Preparation time: 10 minutes

Cooking time: 30 minutes

Servings: 4

Ingredients:

- 1 Tablespoon Olive Oil
- 1 Red Bell Pepper, Diced
- 1 Sweet Onion, Diced
- 2 Tomatoes, Chopped
- 1 Teaspoon Vegan Worcestershire Sauce
- 1 Teaspoon chili Powder
- ½ Teaspoon Thyme
- ½ Teaspoon Garlic Powder
- Sea Salt & Black Pepper to Taste
- 1 Cup Black Eyed Peas, Rinsed
- 3 ¼ Cups Vegetable Stock
- 1 Cup Peas, Frozen
- 3 Cups Kale, Fresh & Chopped
- 2 Cups Brown Rice, Cooked

Directions:

1. Press sauté and set I tot low and then add the oil.
2. Once it's hot cook the bell pepper and onion for three minutes, stirring often.
3. Turn off sauté and then add in the chili powder, tomatoes, vegan Worcestershire sauce, garlic powder, salt, pepper, garlic powder, black eyed peas and stock.
4. Seal the lid, and cook on high pressure for twenty minutes.
5. Use a natural pressure release for twenty minutes and then finish with a quick release.
6. Add the frozen peas, kale and rice, and stir well.

Vegan Spec. Salad

Preparation time: 10 minutes

Cooking time: 30 minutes

Servings: 4

Ingredients:

- 1 Eggplant, Sliced
- 2 Zucchini, Sliced
- 1 Tablespoon Olive Oil
- 3 Tomatoes, Sliced
- 2 Cups Water

Directions:

1. Pour your water in, and then get out a baking dish.
2. Layer your eggplant, tomatoes and zucchini until you run out of ingredients.
3. Spritz with olive oil, and then add in your trivet.
4. Put the baking dish on top of the trivet.
5. Secure the lid, and cook on high pressure for ten minutes.
6. Use a natural release before serving.

Moo Goo Gai Pan

Preparation time: 10 minutes

Cooking time: 40 minutes

Servings: 4

Ingredients:

Marinade:

- 2 Tablespoons Soy Sauce, Lite
- 2 Tablespoons Vegetable Stock
- 1 Tablespoon Sesame Oil
- 1 Clove Garlic, Minced
- ½ Inch Ginger, Fresh, Peeled & Grated

Stir Fry:

- 14 Ounces Firm Tofu, Pressed Overnight & Cubed
- 1 Tablespoon Sesame Oil
- 8 Ounces White Mushrooms, Sliced
- 1 Carrot, Julienned
- 1 Cup Sugar Snap Peas, Rinsed & Trimmed
- 1 Clove Garlic, Minced
- 1 Cup Vegetable Stock

- 1 Inch Piece Ginger, Peeled & Grated
- 2 Tablespoons Soy Sauce
- 8 Ounces Water Chestnuts, Canned, Sliced & Drained
- 8 Ounces Bamboo Shoots, Canned & Drained
- 1 Tablespoon Cornstarch
- 1/3 Cup Hot Water Cooked Noodles for Serving

Directions:

1. Start by making your marinade by whisking all ingredients together, and then add in your tofu.
2. Allow it to marinate for thirty minutes.
3. Press sauté and set it to low, and then add in the oil.
4. Once it's hot add in the marinated tofu, and cook for ten minutes.
5. Remove your tofu and place it to the side.
6. Turn your instant pot off of sauté and then add in your carrot, garlic, ginger, snap peas, mushrooms, stock, soy sauce, bamboo shoots and water chestnuts.
7. Stir well.
8. Press sauté and select low once more, and cover your pot using a tempered glass lid, letting it simmer for five minutes.
9. Stir often.
10. Get out a bowl and whisk the water and cornstarch together to make a slurry.

11. Add it to the pot, and then simmer while uncovered for five minutes.

12. Serve over noodles.

Cauliflower Red Curry

Preparation time: 10 minutes

Cooking time: 30 minutes

Servings: 4

Ingredients:

- 2 Tablespoons Red Curry Paste
- 1 Teaspoon Garlic Powder
- 1 Cup Water
- 14 Ounces Coconut Milk, Canned & Full Fat
- Sea Salt & Black Pepper to Taste
- ¼ Teaspoon Chili Powder
- ½ Teaspoon Ginger
- 1 Bell Pepper, Sliced Thin
- 1 Cauliflower Head, Chopped
- 14 Ounces Tomatoes with Liquid, Canned & Diced Cooked
- Rice for Serving

Directions:

1. Stir your red curry paste, garlic powder, salt, ginger, onion powder chili powder, water, and coconut milk together in your instant pot.
2. Throw in your cauliflower, tomatoes and bell pepper next.
3. Stir well, and then seal the lid.
4. Cook on high pressure for two minutes.
5. Use a quick release, and stir well before serving over rice.

Lasagna Soup

Preparation time: 10 minutes

Cooking time: 40 minutes

Servings: 4

Ingredients:

- 2 Tablespoons Olive Oil
- 1 Onion, Diced
- 1 Clove Garlic, Diced
- 2 Teaspoons Oregano
- 1 Teaspoon Rosemary
- ¾ Teaspoons Red Pepper Flakes
- ½ Teaspoon Sea Salt, Fine
- 2 Tomatoes, Chopped
- 1 Cube Vegetable Bouillon
- 1 Bay Leaf
- 10 Lasagna Noodles, Broken
- 2/3 Cup Red Sauce
- 6 Cups Water Sea
- Salt & Black Pepper to Taste
- Basil, Fresh for Garnish

- Shredded Vegan Cheese for Garnish

Directions:

1. Press sauté, and then add in the oil.
2. Heat until it begins to shimmer, and then throw in your onion.
3. Cook for three minutes before tossing in your garlic.
4. Cook for another minute, and stir often to keep it from burning.
5. Add the rosemary, red pepper flakes, oregano, salt, bouillon cube, tomatoes, bay leaf, noodles, water and red sauce.
6. Stir well, and make sure that your noodles are completely submerged.
7. Seal the lid, and then cook on high pressure for four minutes.
8. Use a natural pressure release for ten minutes before finishing with a quick release.
9. Discard the bay leaf, and season with salt and pepper before serving garnished with basil and vegan cheese.

Apple Cider Vinegar Main:

- 8 Ounces Stir Fry Noodles
- 2 Cups Pea Pods, Fresh
- 4 Carrots, Julienned
- 2 Red Peppers, Sliced
- ½ Red Onion, Sliced

Toppings:

- Cilantro Peanuts Lime Juice

Directions:

1. Start by combining all of your sauce ingredients in your instant pot and then press sauté.
2. Once it starts to boil, stir the noodles in. allow it to simmer for three minutes, but make sure to stir often.
3. Turn the instant pot off of sauté.
4. Then seal the lid, and cook on high pressure for a minute.
5. Use a quick release, and then combine your vegetables.
6. Mix well and garnish before serving warm.

Beets, Edamame & Mixed Green Salad

Preparation Time: 10 minutes

Cooking Time: 0 minute

Serving: 1

Ingredients:

- 2 cups mixed greens
- ½ raw beet, peeled and shredded
- 1 cup shelled edamame, thawed
- 1 tablespoon red wine vinegar
- 1 tablespoon fresh cilantro, chopped
- 2 teaspoons extra-virgin olive oil
- Pepper to taste

Directions:

1. Place the mixed greens in a food container.
2. Top with shredded beets and edamame.
3. In a glass jar with lid, mix the rest of the Ingredients.

4. Refrigerate the salad and drizzle with the dressing when ready to eat.

Black Bean & Corn Salad

Preparation Time: 15 minutes

Cooking Time: 0 minute

Servings: 4

Ingredients:

- 2 tablespoons olive oil
- ¼ cup lime juice
- ¼ cup fresh cilantro, chopped
- Salt and pepper to taste
- 2 cups red cabbage, shredded
- 2 ¼ cups corn kernels
- ⅓ cup pine nuts, toasted
- 30 oz. canned black beans, rinsed and drained
- 1 tomato, diced
- ½ cup red onion, minced

Directions:

1. In a glass jar with lid, blend the oil, lime juice, cilantro, salt and pepper.

2. In a food container, arrange the red cabbage, topped with the rest of the Ingredients.

3. Cover and refrigerate until ready to serve.

4. Drizzle with dressing before serving.

Cheese Paste

Preparation Time: 30minutes

Ingredients:

- 1/2 cup chopped red peppers
- 2 tbsp water
- 2 tbsp Nutritional yeast
- 2 tbsp freshly squeezed lemon juice
- 3/4 teaspoon Himalayan crystal salt or sea salt
- 1/4 tsp paprika powder
- 1/4 teaspoon smoked paprika powder
- 1/4 teaspoon turmeric powder
- 2 large pinches of cayenne
- 1 cup finely ground cashews

Directions:

1. Combine red peppers, water, yeast, lemon juice, salt, paprika powder, smoked paprika, turmeric powder, cayenne pepper and finely ground cashews in a blender.
2. Mix until smooth.

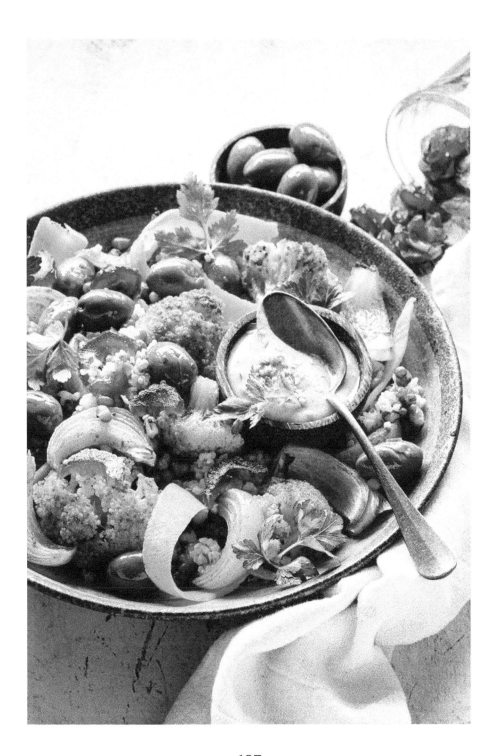

Lightning Source UK Ltd.
Milton Keynes UK
UKHW020705130521
383649UK00005B/93

9 781802 772647